Six Minutes Meal

Relish the Speed: Delectable Feasts in Only Six Minutes!"

Ford Miller

Copyright © 2023 by Ford Miller

Table of Contents: Six-Minute Meals

Introduction

In a comfortable little house settled in the midst of the moving slopes, carried on with an individual named Alex, who had a surprising ability for culinary wizardry. Alex had forever been interested by the specialty of cooking, continually looking for new recipes and strategies to make heavenly dishes. Their enthusiasm for food was matched exclusively by their adoration for writing.

One bright morning, as the brilliant beams of the sun sifted through the bungalow windows, Alex wound up engaged in a charming book called "The Quick Kitchen: Culinary Marvels in Minutes." This mystical book contained a variety of recipes, each encouraging to convey heavenly dinners in only minutes.

As Alex flipped through the pages, their eyes extended with energy. They coincidentally found a recipe for a connoisseur dinner that grabbed their eye — a heavenly blend of spice cooked chicken, buttered vegetables, and feathery pureed potatoes. The greatest aspect? The whole feast could be ready in only six minutes!

Alex's heart dashed with expectation as they accumulated the important fixings. They briskly preheated the stove and slashed the energetic vegetables with quick accuracy. Looking at the book, they noticed the specific estimations and marinated the chicken with a great mix of flavors.

The commencement started as Alex adhered to the directions with steadfast concentration. They sautéed the vegetables, their faculties buzzing with the tempting smell that filled the kitchen. In the mean time, the chicken sizzled in the stove, turning a lovely brilliant tone.

Time appeared to both stretch and therapist as Alex moved with rehearsed effortlessness. The potatoes were bubbled and squashed flawlessly, their cushy surface promising a wonderful chomp. With minutes left at work, they plated the vegetables, the cooked chicken, and a liberal spot of pureed potatoes, organizing the dinner with a bit of creative artfulness.

As the last seconds ticked away, Alex wondered about the work of art they had made in record time. A feeling of achievement washed over them, an acknowledgment that their affection for writing and culinary ability had crashed in an agreeable ensemble. They raised their creation to their lips and enjoyed each chomp, delighting in the wonderful flavors that moved on their sense of taste.

Expression of Alex's striking accomplishment spread like quickly through the town. Individuals from all over rushed to their cabin, anxious to observe the enchantment of culinary speculative chemistry unfurl right in front of them. Alex turned into a nearby legend, enamoring hearts and taste buds with their capacity to plan remarkable feasts in only minutes, all through the force of perusing.

As the years passed, Alex kept on investigating the universe of cooking and writing, always interlacing their two interests. Their house turned into a safe-haven of motivation, where hopeful cooks and book darlings looked for direction and tracked down comfort in the common appreciation for both gastronomy and the composed word.

Thus, the story of Alex, the culinary bibliophile, turned into a demonstration of the surprising marvels that can be accomplished when energy, information, and a dash of enchantment mix together to make something genuinely remarkable.

In our speedy world, carving out opportunity to set up a nutritious and fulfilling dinner can frequently be a test. The requests of work, school, and different obligations can pass on us with brief period and energy to devote to cooking. In any case, there is an answer that offers comfort without settling for less on taste or wellbeing: Six-Minute Feasts.

Six-Minute Feasts are the exemplification of effectiveness in the kitchen. They are painstakingly created recipes intended to be ready and cooked in only six minutes, giving an answer for those looking for a fast and flavorful dinner without forfeiting quality. With insignificant time venture, you can partake in various tasty dishes that take special care of various preferences and dietary inclinations.

The idea of Six-Minute Dinners goes past simple speed; it additionally underscores effortlessness and openness. These dinners are intended to be not difficult to follow, with clear guidelines and insignificant fixings. Regardless of whether you're a beginner in the kitchen, you'll find yourself fit for preparing a wonderful feast quickly.

One of the incredible benefits of Six-Minute Dinners is their adaptability. They envelop a great many foods, including global flavors and local claims to fame. From Italian pasta dishes to Asian sautés, Mexican tacos to Mediterranean servings of mixed greens, you'll track down a variety of choices to suit your culinary cravings. Whether you favor meat-based dishes or are following a veggie lover, vegetarian, or without gluten diet, there are Six-Minute Dinners to take care of your requirements.

The accentuation on nourishment is one more vital part of Six-Minute Dinners. While they focus on proficiency, these dinners are painstakingly adjusted to give a healthy mix of proteins, carbs, sound fats, and fundamental nutrients and minerals. They consolidate new fixings, guaranteeing that you can partake in a feeding feast without settling for less on wellbeing.

Past their efficient advantages and healthy benefit, Six-Minute Dinners can likewise be an extraordinary method for exploring different avenues regarding new flavors and extend your culinary collection. They acquaint you with various cooking strategies, fixing mixes, and extraordinary flavors, permitting you to encounter the delight of different foods in the solace of your own home.

All in all, Six-Minute Dinners offer a helpful and tasty answer for those looking for fast, simple, and fulfilling feasts. They are intended to be cooked in only six minutes, making them ideal for occupied people or anybody hoping to limit their time in the kitchen. With their flexibility, sustenance, and culinary investigation potential, Six-Minute Dinners give an exceptional harmony among comfort and taste. So why not leave on a culinary experience and find the miracles of Six-Minute Feasts? Your taste buds and occupied timetable will much obliged!

Purpose of Six–Minute Meals

The motivation behind six-minute dinners is to give people a fast, helpful, and sound choice for their feasts. In the present quick moving world, individuals frequently set aside themselves tied for opportunity and battling to offset their bustling timetables with good dieting propensities. Six-minute dinners plan to address this test by offering an answer that is both time-proficient and nutritious.

Time Proficiency: The main role of six-minute dinners is to save time. The idea spins around setting up a feast in no less than six minutes or less, making it ideal for people who are continually in a hurry or have restricted chance to cook. By smoothing out the cooking system and zeroing in on fast and basic recipes, six-minute dinners permit individuals to partake in a custom made feast without investing unreasonable energy in the kitchen.

Comfort: One more critical reason for six-minute dinners is accommodation. These feasts are intended to be effectively open and require negligible exertion concerning readiness and cooking. They are much of the time based on pre-bundled or pre-arranged fixings that can be immediately collected or warmed. This comfort factor requests to people who might not have progressed culinary abilities or who essentially need an issue free choice for their dinners.

Wellbeing and Sustenance: While accommodation and time productivity are fundamental parts of six-minute dinners, they likewise focus on wellbeing and nourishment. In spite of the normal discernment that quick dinners are innately unfortunate, six-minute feasts center around consolidating healthy fixings, adjusted sustenance, and piece control. They underscore utilizing new produce, lean proteins, entire grains, and other supplement rich parts to make balanced and fulfilling feasts. By advancing better choices, six-minute feasts mean to help people in keeping a nutritious eating regimen regardless of their bustling ways of life.

Assortment and Customization: Six-minute feasts are not restricted to a particular food or dietary inclination. They incorporate a large number of recipes, obliging different dietary requirements, including veggie lover, vegetarian, sans gluten, and low-carb choices. This adaptability permits people to redo their feasts in light of their own inclinations, dietary limitations, or wellbeing objectives. By offering a different determination of recipes, six-minute feasts take care of a more extensive crowd and guarantee that everybody can find reasonable choices that line up with their preferences and dietary prerequisites.

Segment Control and Weight The executives: Piece control is a basic piece of the reason behind six-minute feasts. By giving pre-divided fixings and recipes, these dinners urge people to consume proper serving sizes and abstain from indulging. Segment control is critical for weight the board and keeping a solid way of life. Six-minute dinners can assist people with controlling their calorie consumption and foster part mindfulness, supporting their endeavors in accomplishing or keeping a sound weight.

Financial plan Cordial: Six-minute feasts can likewise be a savvy choice for people on a tight spending plan. By zeroing in on basic fixings and limiting waste, these feasts assist with diminishing staple costs. Also, getting ready dinners at home as opposed to depending on takeout or conveyance administrations can set aside cash over the long haul. The moderateness part of six-minute feasts makes them open to a more extensive scope of individuals who might be searching for prudent yet nutritious dinner arrangements.

In synopsis, the motivation behind six-minute dinners is to offer a period effective, helpful, and sound option for people who carry on with occupied existences. By focusing on fast readiness, comfort, sustenance, assortment, segment control, and moderateness, these dinners endeavor to assist people with keeping a reasonable eating routine and pursue better food decisions regardless of their rushed timetables.

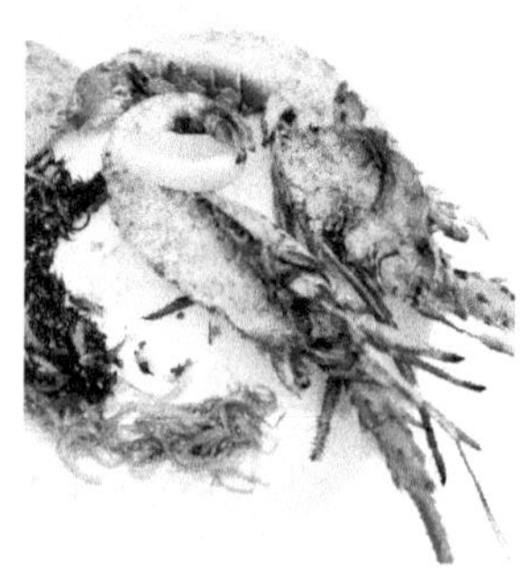

Benefits of Quick and Easy Cooking

In the present high speed world, time has turned into a valuable product. Fast and simple cooking strategies have acquired prominence as they offer various advantages for people and families the same. This thorough substance investigates the upsides of speedy and simple cooking, featuring how it saves time, advances wellbeing, and upgrades imagination in the kitchen.

Efficient:

One of the essential benefits of speedy and simple cooking is the time it saves. Conventional cooking strategies frequently require broad planning and cooking times, which can be difficult for occupied people. With fast and simple recipes, you can essentially lessen the time spent in the kitchen. By using efficient methods, for example, one-pot feasts, sheet skillet suppers, or utilizing kitchen contraptions like strain cookers or slow cookers, you can plan delightful dinners in a negligible portion of the time.

Medical advantages:

In spite of mainstream thinking, fast and simple cooking doesn't be guaranteed to mean forfeiting sustenance. By utilizing new fixings and settling on straightforward cooking techniques, you can in any case make healthy and nutritious feasts. Fast cooking strategies like pan-searing or steaming assist with holding the regular flavors and supplements of the fixings. Furthermore, when you cook at home, you have command over the nature of fixings, segment sizes, and how much salt, sugar, and unfortunate fats utilized in your dinners.

Assortment and innovativeness:

Speedy and simple cooking empowers trial and error and imagination in the kitchen. With a wealth of online assets, cookbooks, and recipe applications accessible, you can undoubtedly track down motivation for speedy feasts that suit your inclinations. This permits you to investigate assorted flavors, cooking styles, and fixings, growing your culinary abilities and sense of taste. Fast cooking likewise empowers you to adjust recipes to suit dietary limitations or food sensitivities, guaranteeing everybody's inclinations are met.

Savvy:

Planning speedy and simple feasts at home can be more savvy than eating out or depending on handled accommodation food varieties. By involving new fixings and cooking in mass, you can set aside cash over the long haul. Moreover, fast cooking strategies frequently require less energy utilization, bringing about decreased service bills. Arranging feasts ahead of time and utilizing extras can likewise limit food waste and stretch your financial plan.

Stress decrease:

Long and complex recipes can be scary and may discourage people from endeavoring to cook at home. Speedy and simple cooking strategies work on the interaction, making it open to even fledgling cooks. By diminishing the pressure related with extended feast arrangement, fast cooking permits you to partake in the experience of preparing and imparting dinners to friends and family.

Improved time with loved ones:

By choosing speedy and simple cooking, you can save important opportunity to enjoy with your loved ones. Rather than going through hours in the kitchen, you can set up a flavorful dinner productively and afterward center around getting a charge out of value time with your friends and family. Speedy cooking can likewise be a great action to include kids or accomplices, cultivating shared encounters and building more grounded connections.

End:

Fast and simple cooking offers many advantages, including time investment funds, further developed wellbeing, improved innovativeness, and cost-viability. By integrating speedy cooking strategies into your culinary collection, you can partake in the accommodation of planning tasty dinners without settling on sustenance or flavor. Whether you're a bustling proficient, a parent, or essentially looking for a more productive method for cooking, embracing speedy and simple cooking strategies can reform your culinary experience and make supper time pleasant, calm, and fulfilling.

Tips for Efficient Meal Preparation

Dinner planning is an important expertise that can assist you with saving time, eat better, and decrease pressure in your everyday existence. By arranging and coordinating your feasts ahead of time, you can guarantee that nutritious and delightful food is promptly accessible, even on your most active days. To capitalize on your dinner planning endeavors, we have ordered a rundown of tips and techniques to assist you with smoothing out your cooking routine and accomplish productive feast readiness.

Plan Your Dinners:

Begin by making a week by week or month to month dinner plan. Think about your dietary requirements, inclinations, and the fixings you as of now have in your storage room. This plan will act as a guide for your feast readiness, guaranteeing you have every one of the essential fixings and lessening the possibilities of somewhat late takeout orders.

Make a Shopping Rundown:

In view of your feast plan, make a thorough shopping list. Assemble comparable fixings to smooth out your shopping experience. Adhere to your rundown when you visit the supermarket to stay away from drive buys and save time.

Bunch Cooking:

Bunch cooking includes planning bigger amounts of food ahead of time and putting away them for sometime in the future. Commit a couple of hours every week to cook staple fixings like grains, proteins, and vegetables. Along these lines, you can make various feasts by basically joining these pre-cooked parts.

Put resources into Feast Prep Compartments:

Put resources into a bunch of top notch feast prep holders in different sizes. These compartments are advantageous for partitioning and putting away your feasts. Pick ones that are microwave-protected and stackable for simple capacity. Having appropriate compartments will assist with keeping up with the newness of your pre-arranged feasts.

Plan Fixings in Mass:

To save time during feast arrangement, wash, cleave, and segment your fixings ahead of time. For instance, cleave vegetables, marinate meats, or cook rice and quinoa quite a bit early. Putting away them appropriately in the fridge or cooler will guarantee they stay new until you are prepared to utilize them.

Sort out Your Kitchen:

Keep your kitchen coordinated and mess free. Organize your cooking tools, pots, and dish in a way that works with simple access. Mark your storeroom things and flavors to rapidly find what you want. An efficient kitchen makes dinner readiness more productive and pleasant.

Use Efficient Apparatuses:

Consider utilizing efficient machines like a sluggish cooker, pressure cooker, or a Moment Pot. These apparatuses can essentially diminish cooking time while as yet delivering tasty feasts. Explore different avenues regarding various recipes and cooking techniques to find what turns out best for you.

Embrace Cooler Dinners:

Cooler dinners are a lifeline when you're in a rush. Get ready enormous clusters of soups, stews, dishes, or sauces, and freeze them in individual or family-sized segments. These dinners can be handily defrosted and warmed, saving you important time during occupied days.

Practice Productive Work processes:

Enhance your cooking interaction by following effective work processes. Begin with undertakings that require longer cooking times or broiler use, and afterward work on different parts while they cook. Perfect as you go to limit post-cooking cleanup time.

Remain Motivated and Adaptable:

Keep a collection of speedy and basic recipes for those occasions when you have restricted time or energy. Look for motivation from cookbooks, online recipe sites, or feast arranging applications. Be adaptable with your feast plan and adjust it as per startling timetable changes or fixing accessibility.

End:

Proficient dinner readiness is a distinct advantage with regards to saving time, decreasing pressure, and keeping a sound eating routine. By executing these tips, you can smooth out your cooking schedule, take advantage of your fixings, and have scrumptious dinners promptly accessible over time. Keep in mind, with just enough preparation and association, dinner arrangement can turn into an agreeable and remunerating part of yours

Chapter 1:Breakfast Recipes

Breakfast is much of the time considered the main feast of the day as it gives the fundamental fuel to launch our morning and keep us stimulated over the course of the day. A nutritious and scrumptious breakfast can establish the vibe for a useful and solid day. Whether you favor something fast and simple or have additional opportunity to set up a good breakfast, the following are a couple of breakfast recipes to move you:

Exemplary Omelet:

Fixings:

2-3 eggs

Salt and pepper to taste

Fillings of your decision (e.g., cheddar, vegetables, ham)

Directions:

Break the eggs into a bowl, season with salt and pepper, and whisk well.

Heat a non-stick dish over medium intensity and empty the beaten eggs into the container.

Permit the eggs to cook briefly until the edges begin to set.

Add your ideal fillings aside of the omelet.

Tenderly crease the opposite side of the omelet over the fillings.

Cook for one more moment until the cheddar liquefies and the omelet is cooked through.

Slide the omelet onto a plate and serve hot.

Short-term Chia Pudding:

Fixings:

1/4 cup chia seeds

1 cup milk (dairy or plant-based)

1 tablespoon sugar (e.g., honey, maple syrup)

Garnishes of your decision (e.g., new organic products, nuts, coconut pieces)

Guidelines:

In a container or bowl, join the chia seeds, milk, and sugar.

Mix well to join and ensure there are no bunches of chia seeds.

Cover the container or bowl and refrigerate for the time being or for no less than 4 hours.

Mix the chia pudding prior to effectively guaranteeing it's equally thickened.

Add your #1 garnishes and partake in a smooth and nutritious chia pudding.

Banana Hotcakes:

Fixings:

1 ready banana

1/2 cup oats

1 egg

1/2 teaspoon baking powder

Touch of salt

1/2 teaspoon vanilla concentrate (discretionary)

Spread or oil for cooking

Fixings of your decision (e.g., new berries, honey, yogurt)

Directions:

In a blender or food processor, mix the banana, oats, egg, baking powder, salt, and vanilla concentrate until smooth.

Heat a non-stick skillet or iron over medium intensity and add a limited quantity of margarine or oil.

Pour little divides of the player onto the dish, shaping flapjacks of your ideal size.

Cook until bubbles structure on a superficial level, then flip the flapjacks and cook the opposite side until brilliant brown.

Serve the banana hotcakes with your number one garnishes and partake in a feathery and normally sweet breakfast treat.

These recipes are only a beginning stage, and you can change them as per your inclinations and dietary necessities. Make sure to focus on a fair and nutritious breakfast to fuel your body and brain for a useful day ahead.

Quick Omelet with Vegetables

A speedy omelet with vegetables is a superb and nutritious dish that can be ready in no time. Loaded with protein, nutrients, and minerals, this flexible feast is ideal for breakfast, lunch, or supper. Whether you're in a hurry or essentially wanting a solid and delightful choice, this omelet recipe makes certain to fulfill your taste buds.

To begin, accumulate the fixings required for your fast omelet. You'll require eggs, vegetables of your decision, for example, chime peppers, onions, mushrooms, spinach, or tomatoes, and a few discretionary flavors like salt, pepper, and spices.

Here is a bit by bit manual for setting up a speedy omelet with vegetables:

Hack the vegetables: Start by washing and slashing your favored vegetables into little, scaled down pieces. This considers even dissemination all through the omelet.

Beat the eggs: Break the ideal number of eggs into a bowl and beat them until the yolks and whites are very much consolidated. You can change the quantity of eggs in light of your craving and serving size.

Sauté the vegetables: Intensity a non-stick skillet or griddle over medium intensity and add a limited quantity of oil or margarine. When the oil is hot, add the hacked vegetables to the skillet and sauté them until they become delicate and somewhat brilliant. This interaction as a rule requires a couple of moments, contingent upon the vegetables you pick.

Season the eggs: While the vegetables are cooking, season the beaten eggs with a spot of salt, pepper, and some other wanted spices or flavors. This step improves the kind of the omelet.

Consolidate eggs and vegetables: When the vegetables are cooked, pour the beaten eggs over them in the skillet. Slant the skillet marginally to guarantee the eggs cover the whole surface and blend well in with the vegetables.

Cook the omelet: Permit the omelet to cook undisturbed for a couple of moments until the base sets. You can marginally lift the edges of the omelet with a spatula to check in the event that the base is cooked. When the base is set, cautiously flip the omelet over utilizing the spatula or by sliding it onto a plate and afterward flipping it back into the container. Cook for an extra little while until the omelet is cooked to your ideal degree of doneness.

Serve and appreciate: Slide the omelet onto a serving plate and trimming with new spices, whenever wanted. It very well may be delighted in with no guarantees or joined by a side of toast, salad, or your number one sauces.

Keep in mind, the excellence of a fast omelet with vegetables lies in its adaptability. You can explore different avenues regarding different vegetable blends, cheeses, or even add cooked meats like ham or chicken for additional protein. Go ahead and tweak the recipe to suit your taste and dietary inclinations.

In a matter of moments by any means, you'll have a delectable and nutritious fast omelet with vegetables fit to be relished. A wonderful and healthy feast can fuel your day and keep you stimulated.

Overnight Chia Pudding

Short-term chia pudding has turned into a famous and helpful breakfast choice for those searching for a solid and flavorful feast to begin their day. This basic yet nutritious dish is made by consolidating chia seeds with fluid and permitting it to thicken for the time being in the cooler.

Chia seeds are minuscule dark or white seeds that come from the Salvia hispanica plant. Regardless of their little size, chia seeds are loaded with supplements. They are an amazing wellspring of fiber, protein, omega-3 unsaturated fats, and different minerals and cancer prevention agents. Furthermore, chia seeds can retain up to multiple times their weight in fluid, shaping a gel-like consistency, which makes them ideal for making a smooth and fulfilling pudding.

Planning for the time being chia pudding is unquestionably simple. To make a fundamental recipe, you will require chia seeds, a fluid of your decision, (for example, almond milk, coconut milk, or dairy milk), and some sugar and flavorings to improve the taste. Just consolidate the chia seeds, fluid, and any ideal increments in a container or a bowl. A few well known increases incorporate vanilla concentrate, cocoa powder, honey, maple syrup, or new natural products.

Whenever you've combined every one of the fixings as one, try to mix well, guaranteeing the chia seeds are equitably dispersed all through the combination. This step is urgent as it forestalls amassing. Then, at that point, cover the compartment and spot it in the cooler short-term or for something like 4-6 hours to permit the chia seeds to retain the fluid and thicken.

By the following morning, you'll have a delicious and smooth chia pudding hanging tight for you. The surface of the chia pudding is like dessert, with a somewhat crunchy surface from the chia seeds. The flavors will have merged together, making a brilliant taste that can be modified as you would prefer.

One of the most engaging parts of for the time being chia pudding is its adaptability. You can try different things with different flavors and garnishes to suit your inclinations. A few well known choices incorporate adding new berries, cut bananas, destroyed coconut, slashed nuts, or a sprinkle of nut margarine on top. The conceivable outcomes are huge, permitting you to make an alternate flavor blend each time you get ready chia pudding.

Aside from being delectable, short-term chia pudding offers a few medical advantages. Chia seeds are wealthy in dietary fiber, which can help processing, advance a sensation of totality, and assist with managing glucose levels. The omega-3 unsaturated fats in chia seeds add to heart wellbeing and lessen aggravation in the body. Moreover, chia seeds are without gluten, making chia pudding reasonable for people with gluten responsive qualities or those following a sans gluten diet.

Whether you're searching for a speedy and simple breakfast choice or a wonderful and sound treat, short-term chia pudding is a phenomenal decision. With its straightforwardness, flexibility, and wholesome advantages, this superb dish has procured its place as a dearest number one among wellbeing cognizant people and food lovers the same. Check it out and partake in a magnificent and supporting treat to launch your day!

Toasted Avocado and Egg Sandwich

The Toasted Avocado and Egg Sandwich is a flavorful and nutritious breakfast choice that consolidates the smoothness of avocado, the protein-pressed decency of eggs, and the fantastic mash of toasted bread. This heavenly creation has acquired fame as of late because of its flavor, straightforwardness, and medical advantages.

To make a Toasted Avocado and Egg Sandwich, you'll require a couple of essential fixings: ready avocados, new eggs, bread cuts of your decision, and a few discretionary increments like spices, flavors, or sauces to upgrade the flavor. Here is a bit by bit manual for creating this magnificent sandwich:

Assemble the fixings: Begin by social event ready avocados that are delicate however not excessively soft. You'll maintain that they should be not difficult to spread on the bread.

Additionally, select new eggs and your favored sort of bread, like entire wheat, sourdough, or multigrain.

Set up the avocado spread: Cut the avocados down the middle the long way and eliminate the pit. Scoop out the tissue into a bowl and squash it with a fork until it arrives at a smooth and spreadable consistency. You can add a spot of salt, dark pepper, or even a press of lime or lemon juice to upgrade the taste.

Cook the eggs: There are different ways of cooking eggs for this sandwich. You can settle on broiled eggs, fried eggs, or even a poached egg on the off chance that you like. Cook the eggs to your ideal degree of doneness, remembering that the runny yolk can add additional richness to the sandwich.

Toast the bread: Take the bread cuts and toast them to your inclination. You can utilize a toaster oven, toaster, or a burner container to accomplish a fresh surface. Toasting the bread adds a delightful crunch and keeps it from becoming saturated when joined with the avocado and eggs.

Gather the sandwich: Take one cut of toasted bread and spread a liberal measure of the squashed avocado on it. Put the cooked eggs on top of the avocado spread. You can decide to cut the eggs or keep them entire, contingent upon your inclination. Add any extra flavors or toppings, like a sprinkle of salt and pepper, hot sauce, or new spices.

Complete the sandwich: Require the second cut of toasted bread and put it on top of the egg layer, making a sandwich. Delicately press it down to assist the fixings with merging together.

Partake in your creation: Your Toasted Avocado and Egg Sandwich is presently fit to be relished. You can serve it right away, cut it down the middle for more straightforward taking care of, or enclose it by material paper or foil for a versatile breakfast choice.

This sandwich offers an agreeable mix of flavors and surfaces. The smooth avocado gives sound fats and fiber, while the eggs convey a protein lift to keep you stimulated over the course of the morning. The toasted bread adds a wonderful crunch and goes about as a tough vessel for the fillings.

Go ahead and alter your sandwich by adding additional fixings like cut tomatoes, fresh bacon, mixed greens, or cheddar. The potential outcomes are inestimable, permitting you to fit the sandwich as you would prefer inclinations and dietary requirements.

Whether you appreciate it as a fast breakfast at home or pack it for an in a hurry feast, the Toasted Avocado and Egg Sandwich is a great choice that joins straightforwardness, taste, and healthful advantages in each nibble.

Chapter 2:Lunch Recipes

Lunchtime is an extraordinary chance to refuel and re-energize your energy levels until the end of the day. Whether you're searching for a fast and simple dinner or something more intricate, there are innumerable lunch recipes to fulfill your taste buds. From servings of mixed greens and sandwiches to soups and sautés, here are some delightful lunch recipes to move your noontime feasts.

Mediterranean Plate of mixed greens:

Consolidate new fresh lettuce, delicious tomatoes, cucumbers, red onions, Kalamata olives, and feta cheddar. Shower with a lemon-spice vinaigrette made with olive oil, lemon juice, garlic, and your #1 spices like oregano and parsley. This invigorating and beautiful serving of mixed greens isn't just loaded with nutrients and minerals yet in addition offers an explosion of Mediterranean flavors.

Caprese Sandwich:

Layer cuts of ready tomatoes, mozzarella cheddar, and new basil leaves on a roll or crusty bread. Sprinkle with balsamic coating or olive oil and season with salt and pepper. This exemplary Italian sandwich is an ideal mix of smooth cheddar, tart tomatoes, and sweet-smelling basil.

Chicken Caesar Wrap:

Barbecue or cook chicken bosom and cut it into slender strips. In a tortilla wrap, spread Caesar dressing, add the chicken, romaine lettuce, and ground Parmesan cheddar. Roll it up firmly and cut into reduced down pieces. This handheld wrap is a helpful and delightful choice for a protein-pressed lunch.

Tomato Basil Soup:

Sauté onions and garlic in olive oil until clear. Add new tomatoes, vegetable or chicken stock, and a small bunch of new basil leaves. Stew until the tomatoes are delicate, then mix the combination until smooth. Season with salt, pepper, and a touch of sugar whenever wanted. Present with a side of hard bread for a soothing and fulfilling lunch.

Asian Pan-seared Noodles:

Cook your selection of noodles, like rice noodles or udon noodles, as indicated by the bundle guidelines. In a hot wok or skillet, pan sear your number one vegetables like chime peppers, carrots, broccoli, and snap peas. Add the cooked noodles and throw them with a sauce made of soy sauce, sesame oil, ginger, garlic, and a dash of honey. Sprinkle with sesame seeds and slashed green onions for an Asian-motivated lunch choice.

Quinoa Salad:

Cook quinoa and let it cool. In a bowl, join the quinoa with diced vegetables like ringer peppers, cucumbers, cherry tomatoes, and avocado. Add new spices like cilantro or parsley, and throw everything with a fiery dressing made of olive oil, lemon juice, Dijon mustard, and salt. This protein-stuffed salad is a nutritious and filling lunch decision.

Keep in mind, these are only a couple of lunch recipe thoughts to kick you off. Go ahead and tweak them in view of your inclinations and dietary limitations. Whether you seriously love vegan dishes, lean proteins, or dynamic flavors, there's a lunch recipe out there that will fulfill your desires and keep you empowered over the course of the day.

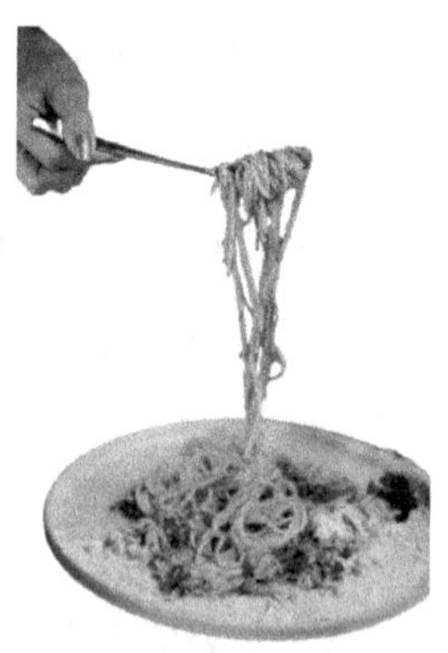

Mediterranean Chickpea Salad

Mediterranean Chickpea Salad is a heavenly and reviving dish that exhibits the energetic flavors and fixings normally tracked down in Mediterranean cooking. Loaded with protein, fiber, and different supplements, this salad isn't just solid yet additionally staggeringly fulfilling.

The star element of this salad is chickpeas, otherwise called garbanzo beans. Chickpeas are a staple in Mediterranean cooking and give a good and nutty base for the serving of mixed greens. They are a brilliant wellspring of plant-based protein and fiber, making them a nutritious expansion to any dinner.

To set up the Mediterranean Chickpea Salad, begin by flushing and depleting a container of chickpeas. Place the chickpeas in a blending bowl and add a liberal measure of hacked new vegetables. Conventional Mediterranean vegetables, for example, cucumber, tomato, ringer peppers, and red onion work superbly in this serving of mixed greens. These vegetables add a reviving crunch and an eruption of variety.

Then, consolidate a small bunch of cleaved new spices like parsley, mint, or cilantro. The spices contribute a dynamic flavor that supplements different fixings and gives the serving of mixed greens its unmistakable Mediterranean taste. Go ahead and change the spice blend in light of your own inclination.

To upgrade the plate of mixed greens' flavors, add disintegrated feta cheddar or tart olives. Feta cheddar adds a rich and pungent component, while olives give a briny and vigorous taste. The two fixings add to the general Mediterranean embodiment of the serving of mixed greens.

For the dressing, whisk together olive oil, lemon juice, garlic, salt, and pepper. This basic yet tasty dressing integrates every one of the fixings and adds a tart and lively component.

Pour the dressing over the plate of mixed greens and throw tenderly to guarantee each fixing is covered.

At long last, let the plate of mixed greens sit in the cooler for around 30 minutes to permit the flavors to merge together. This chilling time likewise permits the chickpeas to retain a portion of the dressing, improving their taste and surface.

At the point when prepared to serve, you can partake in the Mediterranean Chickpea Salad as a light and fulfilling feast all alone or as a side dish close by barbecued chicken, fish, or sheep. It's likewise a fabulous choice for picnics, potlucks, or as a reviving serving of mixed greens for summer get-togethers.

The Mediterranean Chickpea Salad pleases the taste buds as well as offers a plenty of medical advantages. Chickpeas give a decent wellspring of plant-based protein and fiber, advancing satiety and helping with processing. The new vegetables and spices are plentiful in nutrients, minerals, and cancer prevention agents, supporting by and large prosperity.

All in all, the Mediterranean Chickpea Salad is a delightful and nutritious dish that embodies the quintessence of Mediterranean cooking. A flexible serving of mixed greens can be delighted in on different events, and its energetic flavors and healthy fixings make it a #1 among those looking for a sound and scrumptious dinner.

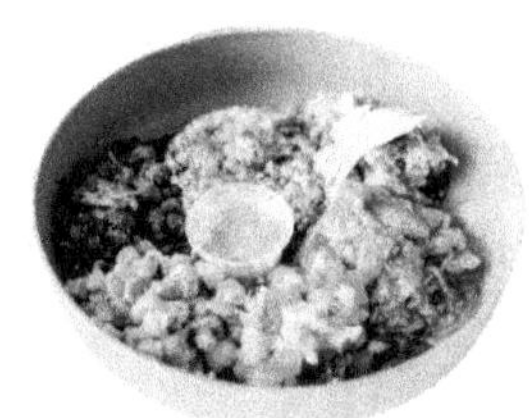

Tuna and White Bean Wrap

Fish and White Bean Wrap is a delectable and nutritious dinner choice that consolidates the kinds of fish, white beans, and different new fixings. It's an ideal decision for those searching for a fast and simple lunch or supper that is loaded with protein, fiber, and sound fats.

To make a Fish and White Bean Wrap, you will require the accompanying fixings:

1 jar of fish, depleted

1 cup of cooked white beans, (for example, cannellini or naval force beans)

1/4 cup of diced red onion

1/4 cup of diced celery

1/4 cup of diced red chime pepper

1/4 cup of diced cucumber

2 tablespoons of hacked new parsley

2 tablespoons of lemon juice

2 tablespoons of olive oil

Salt and pepper to taste

Entire wheat tortillas or wraps

Here is a bit by bit manual for making a Fish and White Bean Wrap:

In a medium-sized bowl, consolidate the depleted fish, cooked white beans, red onion, celery, red chime pepper, cucumber, and cleaved parsley. Blend well to consolidate.

In a different little bowl, whisk together the lemon juice, olive oil, salt, and pepper to make a basic dressing.

Pour the dressing over the fish and white bean blend and throw tenderly to uniformly cover every one of the fixings.

Take an entire wheat tortilla or wrap and spoon a liberal measure of the fish and white bean combination onto the focal point of the tortilla.

Crease the sides of the tortilla over the filling, then roll it up firmly from one finish to the next to make a wrap.

Rehash the interaction with the leftover tortillas and filling.

When every one of the wraps are ready, you can either serve them right away or wrap them firmly in saran wrap and refrigerate for later utilization.

Fish and White Bean Wraps can be delighted in as an independent dinner or matched with a side plate of mixed greens or some new natural product for a balanced and fulfilling feast. They are adaptable and can be modified by your taste inclinations. You can add extra fixings like avocado cuts, cherry tomatoes, or destroyed lettuce to improve the flavor and surface.

Not exclusively are Fish and White Bean Wraps scrumptious, however they are likewise a sound choice. Fish is a great wellspring of lean protein, omega-3 unsaturated fats, and different fundamental supplements. White beans are loaded with fiber, protein, and other significant supplements like iron and folate. This mix makes the wrap a filling and nutritious decision.

Whether you're searching for a fast lunch to take to work, a basic supper choice, or a nutritious bite, Fish and White Bean Wraps are a heavenly and fulfilling decision that is not difficult to plan and appreciate.

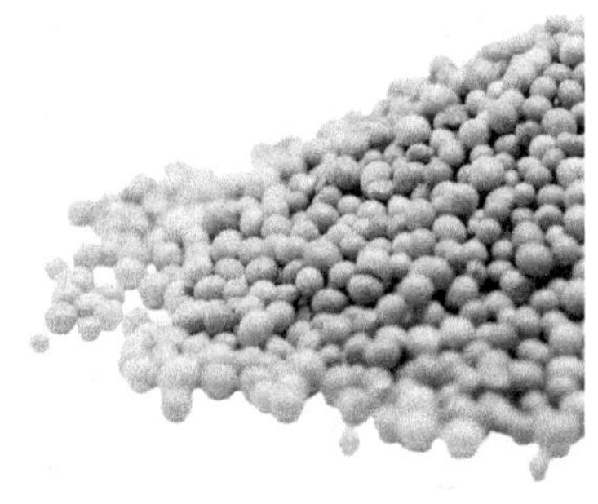

Caprese Pasta Salad

Caprese pasta salad is a magnificent and invigorating dish that joins the kinds of an exemplary Caprese salad with the generosity of pasta. It is an ideal choice for those looking for a light and fulfilling feast throughout the late spring months or at whatever point you desire an explosion of Mediterranean flavors.

The groundwork of Caprese pasta salad is normally cooked pasta, for example, fusilli or penne, albeit different sorts can be utilized relying upon individual inclination. The cooked pasta is then thrown with different fixings that complete one another impeccably.

One of the principal parts of Caprese pasta salad is new tomatoes. Ready, delicious tomatoes add an explosion of pleasantness and causticity to the dish. Cherry tomatoes or diced Roma tomatoes function admirably. To upgrade the flavor, it is fitting to utilize plant matured tomatoes when they are in season.

One more fundamental component of Caprese pasta salad is new mozzarella cheddar. The mozzarella is generally cut into little 3D squares or attacked scaled down pieces and dispersed all through the plate of mixed greens. The velvety and gentle kind of the cheddar coordinates magnificently with the tart tomatoes.

To draw out the dynamic flavors, new basil leaves are an unquestionable necessity. Basil adds a fragrant and sweet-smelling note to the serving of mixed greens. Tear the basil leaves into more modest pieces or chiffonade them (fold the leaves firmly and cut into dainty strips) to deliver their magnificent smell.

The dressing for Caprese pasta salad is ordinarily light and straightforward, permitting the kinds of the fixings to sparkle. Additional virgin olive oil is a staple in this dish, as it adds lavishness and a fruity feeling. A sprinkle of balsamic vinegar or a press of lemon juice can be added to light up the flavors and give an inconspicuous tartness.

Salt and newly ground dark pepper are fundamental for preparing the serving of mixed greens. These basic fixings assist with adjusting the flavors and improve the general taste.

Caprese pasta salad can be modified to suit individual inclinations and dietary limitations. For a heartier choice, you can add barbecued chicken or shrimp to the serving of mixed greens. Then again, you can integrate different vegetables like cut cucumbers, cooked red peppers, or olives to mix it up.

Whether filled in as a side dish or an independent feast, Caprese pasta salad is a flexible and swarm satisfying choice. It very well may be delighted in at picnics, potlucks, grills, or as a light lunch or supper choice. The blend of new fixings and Mediterranean flavors makes it an invigorating and fulfilling dish for warm climate get-togethers or any time you need to relish the flavor of summer.

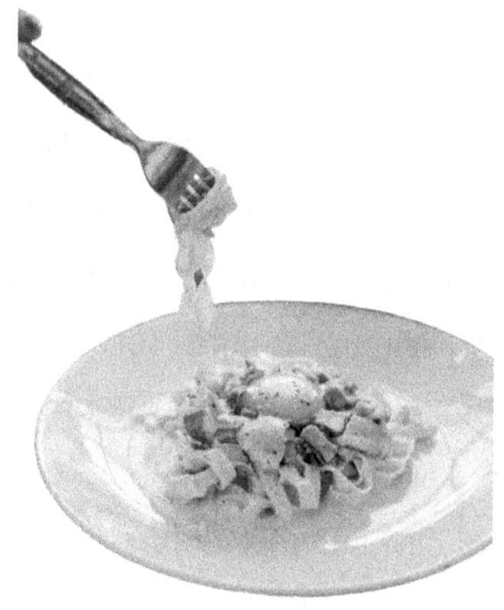

Chapter 3:Dinner Recipes

Supper time is a superb chance to accumulate with friends and family and partake in a tasty feast together. Whether you're cooking for yourself, your family, or facilitating a supper get-together, having a collection of supper recipes is fundamental. From soothing works of art to imaginative dishes, the following are a couple of supper recipes to move you:

Exemplary Dish Chicken:

Broil chicken is an immortal supper choice that never disappoints. Season an entire chicken with salt, pepper, and spices of your decision (like rosemary or thyme). Cook it in the stove until the skin is fresh and brilliant, and the meat is succulent and delicate. Present with simmered vegetables and a side of pureed potatoes for a delightful feast.

Spaghetti Bolognese:

This Italian exemplary is a group pleaser and ideal for a family supper. Sauté ground hamburger or a meat substitute with onions, garlic, and diced carrots until seared. Add pureed tomatoes, a sprinkle of red wine, spices (like basil and oregano), and let it stew for some time to foster flavors. Serve the sauce over cooked spaghetti and sprinkle with ground Parmesan cheddar.

Vegan Sautéed food:

For a fast and solid supper, a vegetable pan fried food is a fabulous choice. Heat a few oil in a wok or huge skillet and add your #1 vegetables like chime peppers, broccoli, carrots, and snap peas. Pan sear until fresh delicate and add a sauce made of soy sauce, ginger, garlic, and a hint of honey or maple syrup for pleasantness. Serve over steamed rice or noodles.

Prepared Salmon with Lemon-Dill Sauce:

Salmon isn't just heavenly yet in addition loaded with sound omega-3 unsaturated fats. Season salmon filets with salt, pepper, and a press of lemon juice. Prepare in the broiler until the fish is flaky and cooked through. For the lemon-dill sauce, combine as one Greek yogurt, new dill, lemon zing, salt, and pepper. Serve the heated salmon with the sauce as an afterthought, alongside steamed asparagus or cooked potatoes.

Mexican Enchiladas:

In the event that you're in the state of mind for a few Mexican flavors, enchiladas are a phenomenal decision. Sauté onions and ringer peppers in a skillet, then add cooked chicken or beans for a vegan choice. Fill tortillas with the combination, roll them up, and place them in a baking dish. Pour enchilada sauce over the top, sprinkle with destroyed cheddar, and prepare until effervescent and brilliant. Present with a side of Mexican rice and guacamole.

These are only a couple of instances of supper recipes to kick you off. Go ahead and explore different avenues regarding various fixings, flavors, and cooking styles to make your own particular dishes. Keep in mind, cooking is an inventive flow, so have a great time and partake in the excursion of setting up a tasty supper for you as well as your friends and family.

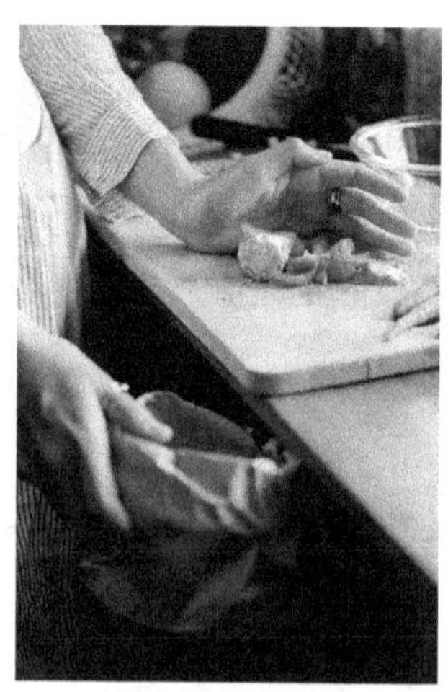

Garlic Shrimp Stir-Fry

Garlic shrimp pan fried food is a delectable and fulfilling dish that unites the delicious kinds of shrimp, the sweet-smelling substance of garlic, and a brilliant combination of new vegetables. This dynamic and tasty sautéed food is simply difficult to plan yet in addition a flexible choice that can be delighted in as an independent feast or served over steamed rice or noodles.

To make a garlic shrimp pan sear, you will require the accompanying fixings:

1 pound (450 grams) of shrimp, stripped and deveined

4 cloves of garlic, minced

1 tablespoon of vegetable oil

1 red ringer pepper, meagerly cut

1 yellow chime pepper, daintily cut

1 little onion, daintily cut

1 cup of snap peas, closes managed

1 cup of broccoli florets

2 tablespoons of soy sauce

1 tablespoon of clam sauce

1 teaspoon of cornstarch, broke up in 2 tablespoons of water

Salt and pepper to taste

Discretionary embellishment: hacked green onions or cilantro

Presently, we should begin with the cooking system:

Heat the vegetable oil in a huge skillet or wok over medium-high intensity.

Add the minced garlic to the hot oil and sauté for around 30 seconds until fragrant, being mindful so as not to consume it.

Add the shrimp to the skillet and cook for 2-3 minutes until they become pink and are cooked through. Eliminate the shrimp from the skillet and put away.

In a similar skillet, add the cut ringer peppers, onion, snap peas, and broccoli. Pan sear the vegetables for 3-4 minutes until they become marginally delicate yet fresh.

In the mean time, in a little bowl, whisk together the soy sauce and clam sauce until very much joined.

Return the cooked shrimp to the skillet and pour the sauce blend over the shrimp and vegetables. Pan sear for an extra 1-2 minutes to guarantee the flavors are all around consolidated.

Mix in the broke up cornstarch blend to thicken the sauce. Keep cooking for one more moment until the sauce has thickened to your ideal consistency.

Season the sautéed food with salt and pepper as per your taste inclinations.

Eliminate the skillet from intensity and enhancement with slashed green onions or cilantro for an additional explosion of newness and variety.

Your garlic shrimp pan fried food is presently fit to be delighted in! Serve it hot as a principal dish or with steamed rice or noodles for a seriously filling dinner. The blend of delicate shrimp, crunchy vegetables, and the powerful kind of garlic will without a doubt fulfill your taste buds and leave you hankering more. This dish offers a superb mix of surfaces and fragrances that make it a group satisfying choice for any event.

Go ahead and modify the recipe by adding different vegetables like carrots, mushrooms, or child corn, contingent upon your inclinations. You can likewise change the fieriness by integrating stew drops or a sprinkle of sriracha sauce in the event that you partake in a touch of intensity.

Whether you're cooking for yourself, your family, or visitors, garlic shrimp sautéed food is a straightforward and flexible recipe that unites the brilliant kinds of the ocean and the fragrant allure of garlic, making it a go-to choice for fish devotees and pan fried food sweethearts the same.

One-Pot Chicken and Rice

One-Pot Chicken and Rice is a tasty and helpful dish that unites delicate chicken, delightful rice, and various spices and flavors in a solitary pot. A delightful and encouraging feast requires insignificant exertion and is ideally suited for occupied weeknights or when you need a problem free cooking experience.

To set one up Pot Chicken and Rice, you'll require the accompanying fixings:

1.5 pounds (680 grams) of boneless, skinless chicken thighs or bosoms

1 cup of long-grain white rice

1 onion, finely hacked

3 cloves of garlic, minced

1 chime pepper, diced

1 carrot, diced

2 cups of chicken stock

1 teaspoon of paprika

1 teaspoon of dried thyme

1/2 teaspoon of dried oregano

1/2 teaspoon of cumin

Salt and pepper to taste

2 tablespoons of olive oil

New parsley or cilantro for embellish (discretionary)

Presently, we should continue with the cooking directions:

Begin via preparing the chicken with salt, pepper, paprika, and cumin. Heat the olive oil in a huge pot or Dutch stove over medium-high intensity.

Add the chicken to the pot and cook until sautéed on the two sides, around 3-4 minutes for each side. Eliminate the chicken from the pot and put it away.

In a similar pot, add the cleaved onion, garlic, ringer pepper, and carrot. Sauté them for a couple of moments until they relax and become fragrant.

Mix in the rice, thyme, and oregano, covering the rice with the tasty combination. Cook for an extra moment to somewhat toast the rice.

Pour in the chicken stock, scratching the lower part of the pot to deliver any carmelized bits. Heat the combination to the point of boiling.

When the fluid is bubbling, lessen the intensity to low and restore the chicken to the pot, nestling it into the rice blend. Cover the pot with a top and let it stew delicately for around 20-25 minutes, or until the rice is cooked and the chicken is delicate.

When the rice is completely cooked, eliminate the pot from intensity and allow it to sit covered for 5 minutes to permit the flavors to merge together.

Cushion the rice with a fork and taste for preparing, changing with salt and pepper if necessary. You can likewise sprinkle some new parsley or cilantro on top for added newness and variety.

Serve the One-Pot Chicken and Rice straightforwardly from the pot, or move it to a serving dish. It coordinates well with a side serving of mixed greens or steamed vegetables.

This magnificent one-pot dinner gives an agreeable blend of protein, starches, and vegetables, making it a balanced dish. The chicken remaining parts succulent and tasty, while the rice retains the delectable stock and fragrant flavors, bringing about a fantastic and soothing plate of food. Partake in the straightforwardness and delectability of One-Pot Chicken and Rice as you appreciate each chomp!

Veggie Stir-Fry with Noodles

Veggie pan sear with noodles is a delectable and solid dish that consolidates the lively kinds of new vegetables with the wonderful surface of noodles. It is a flexible and simple to-create recipe that can be modified to suit your taste inclinations and dietary necessities.

To make a veggie pan sear with noodles, you'll require different beautiful vegetables, for example, ringer peppers, carrots, broccoli, snap peas, and mushrooms. You can likewise add different vegetables like bok choy, zucchini, or cabbage, contingent upon your inclination. The key is to utilize vegetables that cook rapidly and hold their freshness when pan-seared.

Begin by setting up the vegetables. Wash them completely and cut them into scaled down pieces. Heat a wok or a huge skillet over medium-high intensity and add some vegetable oil. When the oil is hot, add the vegetables beginning with the ones that take more time to cook, like carrots and broccoli. Pan sear them for two or three minutes until they start to relax. Then, add the leftover vegetables and proceed with pan-searing for an additional couple of moments until they are marginally delicate yet at the same time hold their crunchiness. You can prepare the vegetables with a touch of salt and pepper or add some minced garlic or ginger for additional character.

While the vegetables are cooking, set up the noodles as indicated by the bundle guidelines. You can utilize any sort of noodles you like, like rice noodles, udon noodles, or soba noodles. Cook them until they are still somewhat firm, then channel and put away.

When the vegetables are cooked as you would prefer, add the cooked noodles to the wok or skillet. Throw everything together delicately, guaranteeing that the noodles get covered with the flavors from the vegetables. Whenever wanted, you can likewise add a pan fried food sauce as of now. A basic sauce produced using soy sauce, sesame oil, and a hint of honey or maple syrup functions admirably. Pan sear for one more little while until everything is all around consolidated.

To serve, move the veggie pan sear with noodles to a serving dish or individual plates. You can decorate it for certain new spices like cilantro or green onions, and sprinkle some toasted sesame seeds for added crunch. In the event that you like it hot, you can add a shower of sriracha or sprinkle some red pepper pieces. Veggie pan sear with noodles is a finished dinner all alone, yet you can likewise serve it with some protein of your decision. Barbecued tofu, tempeh, or seitan make fantastic vegan choices, while cooked shrimp, chicken, or hamburger can be added for meat darlings.

This dish isn't just flavorful, yet it likewise gives a nutritious equilibrium between vegetables and carbs. It's an extraordinary method for integrating more veggies into your eating routine and is reasonable for vegans and vegetarians. Partake in the vivid and delightful decency of veggie pan sear with noodles as a fantastic and healthy feast!

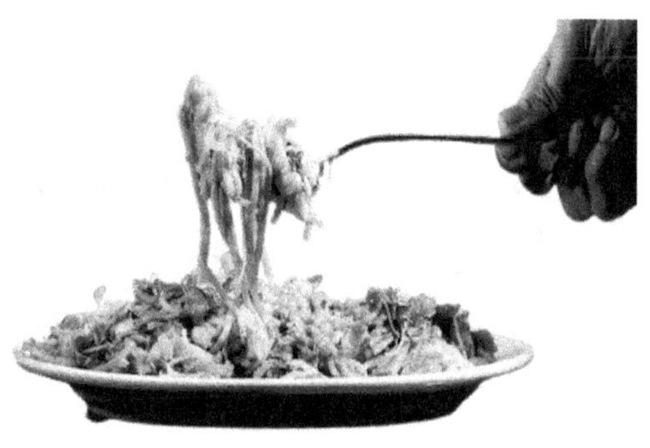

Chapter 4:Snack Recipes

Snacks are a superb and helpful method for fulfilling your desires between feasts. Whether you're searching for a light meal during a film night, a delectable treat for a social occasion, or a delightful choice to fuel your typical working day, nibble recipes offer vast potential outcomes. From appetizing to sweet, here are some delightful nibble thoughts that make certain to stimulate your taste buds:

Guacamole and Veggie Sticks:

Prepare a new clump of guacamole by crushing ready avocados with lime juice, diced tomatoes, red onions, cilantro, and a spot of salt. Serve it with a combination of beautiful veggie sticks like carrots, celery, ringer peppers, and cucumber for a crunchy and sound tidbit.

Natively constructed Popcorn:

Make your film evenings shockingly better with natively constructed popcorn. Heat some oil in an enormous pot, add popcorn pieces, cover, and let them pop over medium intensity. Once finished, season it with dissolved spread and sprinkle with your #1 fixings like ground Parmesan cheddar, bean stew powder, or caramel for a sweet turn.

Caprese Sticks:

Collect small sticks with cherry tomatoes, reduced down mozzarella balls, and new basil leaves. Shower them with balsamic coating or a sprinkle of salt and pepper for a basic yet rich tidbit that is overflowing with flavors.

Greek Yogurt Parfait:

Layer rich Greek yogurt with a variety of new natural products like berries, cut bananas, and diced mango. Finish it off with a sprinkle of granola or cleaved nuts for added surface and partake in this reviving and nutritious tidbit.

Smaller than expected Quiches:

Plan reduced down quiches by whisking together eggs, milk, cheddar, and your selection of fillings like diced ham, sautéed vegetables, or spinach. Empty the combination into lubed biscuit tins and heat until brilliant and set. These little quiches are ideal for parties or as an in and out nibble.

Energy Balls:

Join moved oats, nut margarine, honey, and a blend of nuts, seeds, and dried natural products in a bowl. Fold the combination into little balls and refrigerate until firm. These energy balls are loaded with supplements and make for a speedy and invigorating tidbit on occupied days.

Prepared Yam Fries:

Cut yams into slender wedges, throw them with olive oil, salt, and flavors like paprika or garlic powder. Organize them on a baking sheet and prepare until fresh. These delightful and better options in contrast to ordinary fries make certain to be a hit.

Chocolate-Plunged Strawberries:

Dissolve dull or drain chocolate in a bowl, plunge new strawberries into the liquefied chocolate, and let them cool on a lined baking sheet. When set, enjoy the overpowering blend of succulent strawberries and rich chocolate.

Keep in mind, the universe of nibble recipes is tremendous, and you can constantly get imaginative and explore different avenues regarding various fixings and flavors. Partake during the time spent getting ready and enjoying these great treats at whatever point you want a tasty jolt of energy.

Energy-Boosting Trail Mix

Energy-Supporting Path Blend: The Ideal Nibble for a Functioning Way of life

In the present quick moving world, keeping up with high energy levels over the course of the day is fundamental, particularly for those driving a functioning way of life. Whether you're climbing, cycling, examining, or basically searching for a sound nibble to fuel your day, energy-supporting path blend is the ideal arrangement. Loaded with different supplement rich fixings, this helpful and tasty blend gives a speedy and practical wellspring of energy.

The groundwork of energy-helping trail blend is nuts and seeds. These power-pressed fixings are stacked with sound fats, proteins, and fiber, making them an ideal energy source. Almonds, cashews, pecans, and peanuts are famous decisions because of their rich flavor and dietary advantages. Moreover, integrating seeds like pumpkin, sunflower, and chia seeds adds an additional portion of supplements like omega-3 unsaturated fats, nutrients, and minerals.

Dried organic products are one more significant part of trail blend, offering normal sugars and a variety of fundamental supplements. Choices like raisins, cranberries, blueberries, and apricots give a magnificent explosion of pleasantness as well as supply cell reinforcements, nutrients, and fiber. They add to keeping up with stable glucose levels and give a speedy jolt of energy without the accidents related with refined sugar.

To add a superb crunch and assortment, including entire grain oat, pretzels, or toasted coconut pieces can hoist the path blend insight. These fixings offer carbs for supported energy, while the grain and pretzels give extra surface and flavor. Coconut drops, specifically, give medium-chain fatty oils (MCTs), which are effectively processed by the body and immediately changed over into energy.

For an additional kick, flavors and flavors can be integrated in with the general mish-mash. Cinnamon, nutmeg, and cocoa powder are incredible decisions that improve the taste as well as proposition potential medical advantages. Cinnamon supports balancing out glucose levels, nutmeg gives mitigating properties, and cocoa powder contains cancer prevention agents and mind-set improving mixtures.

Making your own energy-supporting path blend considers customization in view of individual inclinations and dietary limitations. Whether you're following a vegetarian, without gluten, or paleo diet, trail blend can be adjusted to suit your requirements. It additionally empowers segment control, guaranteeing that you consume the perfect proportion of calories and supplements for ideal energy levels.

Energy-supporting path blend is a flexible tidbit that can be delighted in on different events. It fills in as a speedy breakfast choice, a late morning jolt of energy, or a pre-exercise nibble. Its helpful bundling makes it simple to convey in a knapsack or satchel, guaranteeing you have a nutritious and empowering nibble any place you go.

Make sure to store your path blend in an impermeable holder to keep up with newness and boost time span of usability. Furthermore, be aware of piece sizes, as trail blend can be calorie-thick. While it gives a phenomenal wellspring of energy, it is critical to consume it with some restraint.

All in all, energy-supporting path blend is a go-to nibble for people looking for supported energy and a helpful healthful lift. With its blend of nuts, seeds, dried natural products, entire grains, and tasty additional items, it offers an equilibrium of macronutrients and micronutrients. Thus, whether you're setting out on a difficult open air experience or basically need a speedy jolt of energy during a bustling day, go after a modest bunch of energy-helping trail blend and let it power you through your exercises with zeal.

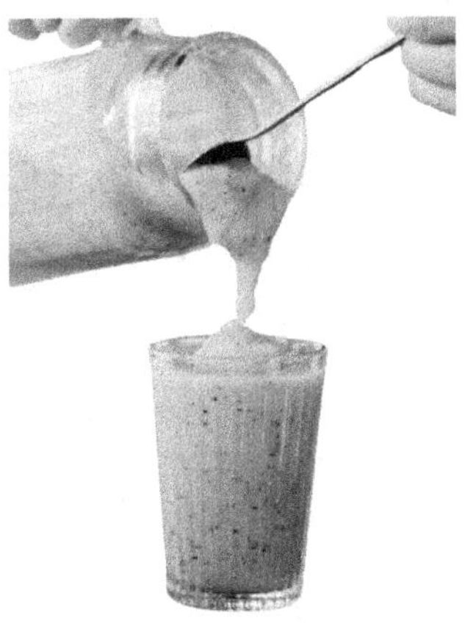

Greek Yogurt with Berries and Granola

Greek Yogurt with Berries and Granola is a tasty and nutritious blend that has become progressively well known as of late. This superb dish offers an ideal equilibrium of rich yogurt, energetic berries, and crunchy granola, making it a delightful and sound choice for breakfast, tidbit, or even treat.

At the core of this dish is Greek yogurt, which contrasts from normal yogurt because of its thicker and creamier surface. Greek yogurt is stressed to eliminate the greater part of the whey, bringing about a higher convergence of protein. It additionally contains less lactose, making it more straightforward to process for those with lactose responsive qualities. Furthermore, Greek yogurt is plentiful in calcium, probiotics, and fundamental nutrients, going with it a fabulous decision for keeping up with stomach wellbeing and supporting generally prosperity.

To improve the flavors and add an eruption of newness, the yogurt is embellished with a grouping of berries. You can browse a wide assortment, like strawberries, blueberries, raspberries, or blackberries, contingent upon your inclination and accessibility. Berries are scrumptious as well as loaded with cell reinforcements, fiber, and fundamental nutrients. They bring a characteristic pleasantness and lively varieties to the dish, making it outwardly engaging.

Finishing the Greek Yogurt with Berries and Granola gathering is the expansion of crunchy granola. Granola is normally produced using a combination of moved oats, nuts, seeds, and sugars like honey or maple syrup, heated until fresh. It adds a superb surface and gives a wonderful smash to each chomp. The blend of the smooth yogurt, delicious berries, and granola makes a great difference of flavors and surfaces.

While setting up this dish, you can collect it in different ways. One choice is to layer the fixings in a bowl or glass, beginning with a liberal scoop of Greek yogurt at the base. Then, add a layer of blended berries, permitting their regular juices to mix with the yogurt. At last, finish it off with a sprinkling of granola, adding a brilliant mash to every spoonful.

On the other hand, you can pick a more adaptable methodology by serving the yogurt, berries, and granola independently, permitting everybody to make their own ideal mix. This is especially advantageous while taking care of individual inclinations or dietary limitations.

Greek Yogurt with Berries and Granola is a flexible dish that can be delighted in whenever of the day. It is an incredible decision for breakfast, giving a nutritious and filling start to your day. On the other hand, it very well may be delighted in as a reviving bite or even as a light sweet after a dinner.

All in all, Greek Yogurt with Berries and Granola is a wonderful and sound dish that joins the richness of Greek yogurt, the normal pleasantness of berries, and the delightful smash of granola. It offers an ideal mix of flavors, surfaces, and fundamental supplements, going with it a phenomenal decision for anybody looking for a healthy and heavenly dinner or bite.

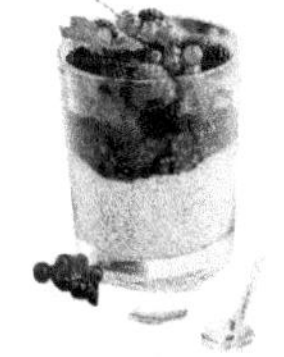

Hummus and Veggie Sticks

Hummus and veggie sticks make for a delightful and nutritious nibble mix that has acquired enormous prevalence as of late. Hummus, a smooth and flavorful plunge produced using pounded chickpeas, mixed with tahini, olive oil, lemon juice, and different flavors, coordinates impeccably with new and crunchy vegetable sticks. This powerful team offers a scope of medical advantages while fulfilling your taste buds.

How about we start with hummus. Beginning from the Center East, hummus has turned into a dearest staple in numerous foods around the world. Chickpeas, the primary fixing, are a fabulous wellspring of plant-based protein, fiber, and fundamental supplements like folate, iron, and manganese. The tahini, produced using sesame seeds, adds sound fats, including omega-3 unsaturated fats, alongside extra protein and fiber. This blend creates hummus a filling and fulfilling plunge that can assist with balancing out glucose levels and advance satiety.

Hummus isn't just nutritious yet additionally inconceivably adaptable. While the exemplary form with chickpeas is generally appreciated, there are various varieties accessible, including simmered red pepper, garlic, sun-dried tomato, and fiery jalapeño. Each flavor adds its own remarkable wind to the smooth base, interesting to various taste inclinations.

Matching hummus with veggie sticks is a fabulous method for integrating more vegetables into your eating regimen. New, brilliant vegetables like carrots, celery, chime peppers, cucumbers, and cherry tomatoes give a variety of nutrients, minerals, and cancer prevention agents. They are low in calories and high in fiber, going with them a superb decision for weight the board and generally wellbeing.

Veggie sticks not just improve the dietary profile of this tidbit yet in addition give a delightful crunch that supplements the perfection of the hummus. The blend of surfaces adds a charming tangible encounter to your nibbling schedule. Besides, the fiber content in vegetables helps processing and adds to a sensation of completion.

One more benefit of hummus and veggie sticks is their accommodation. They are versatile, making them a brilliant choice for in a hurry eating or as a fast and solid starter for social occasions. They require negligible planning and are effectively adaptable in light of individual inclinations and dietary limitations.

All in all, hummus and veggie sticks offer a healthy and delectable nibbling choice. With their rich supplement content, adaptability, and accommodation, they settle on for an optimal decision to fuel your body with fundamental supplements while fulfilling your desires. Whether you appreciate them as a noontime nibble, part of a party platter, or as a backup to a feast, this blend makes certain to charm your taste buds and advance a better way of life.

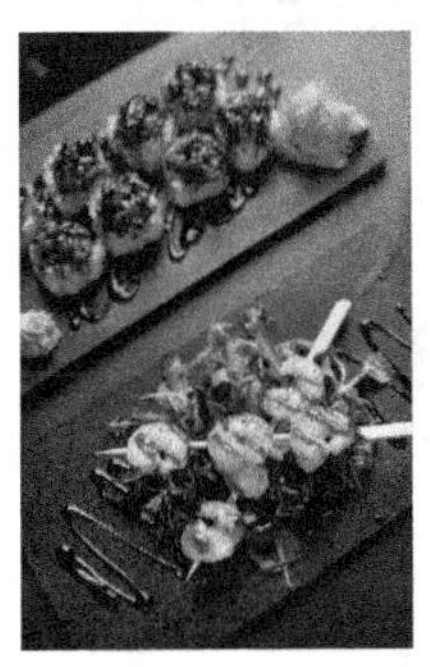

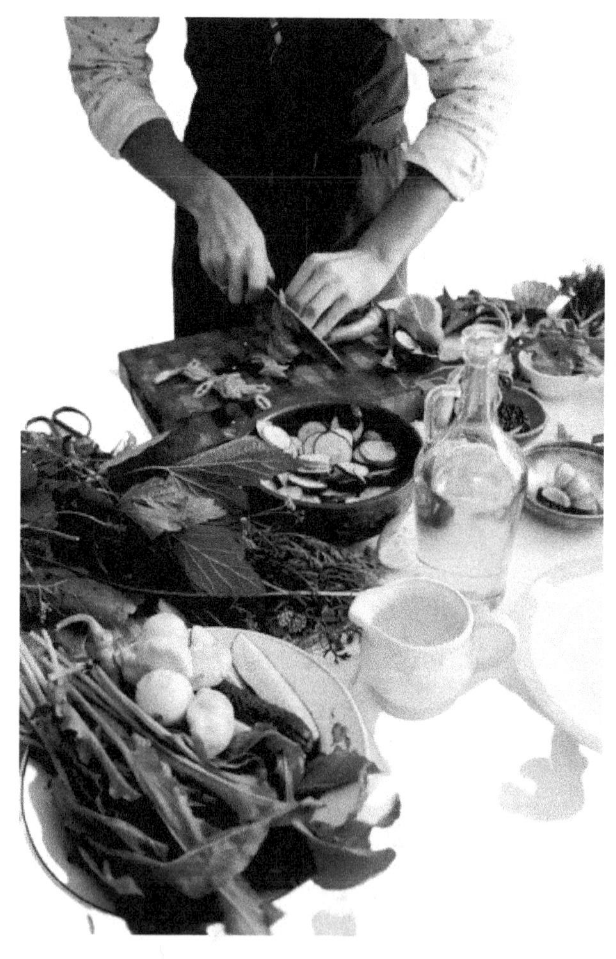

Chapter 5:Dessert Recipes

Dessert are the ideal method for finishing a dinner on a sweet note or fulfill your hankering for something liberal. From exemplary top picks to imaginative manifestations, dessert recipes offer a great many choices to suit each taste. Whether you're a carefully prepared pastry specialist or a fledgling in the kitchen, there's a treat recipe out there for you. How about we investigate some scrumptious and famous pastry recipes that make certain to please your taste buds.

Chocolate Magma Cake:

A work of art and wanton pastry, chocolate magma cake is a rich and gooey treat that will satisfy any chocolate darling. The external layer is a damp chocolate cake, while the middle is loaded up with warm, liquid chocolate. Serve it with a scoop of vanilla frozen yogurt or a spot of whipped cream for an additional hint of extravagance.

Fruity dessert:

Fruity dessert is an immortal pastry that is ideally suited for any event. The flaky hull encases a sweet and tart apple filling, enhanced with cinnamon and nutmeg. Serve it warm with a scoop of vanilla frozen yogurt for a consoling and nostalgic treat.

Crème Brûlée:

Crème brûlée is a velvety and exquisite French sweet that never disappoints. It comprises of a smooth custard base enhanced with vanilla and finished off with a layer of caramelized sugar. Break the caramelized sugar with your spoon to uncover the delicious custard under.

Tiramisu:

Tiramisu is an Italian pastry that consolidates layers of espresso splashed ladyfingers and a rich mascarpone cream. Tidied with cocoa powder on top, this treat is an ideal harmony between flavors and surfaces. It's a group pleaser and an extraordinary make-ahead dessert for evening gatherings.

Strawberry Shortcake:

A light and reviving treat, strawberry shortcake is a brilliant way to exhibit new strawberries. The treat comprises of a rich and brittle shortcake bread roll, finished off with improved strawberries and a touch of whipped cream. It's a brilliant summer treat that is both straightforward and fulfilling.

Chocolate Chip Treats:

Once in a while, nothing beats the exemplary chocolate chip treat. These chewy and tasty treats are stacked with chocolate chips and have a delicate focus with a marginally firm edge. Appreciate them warm with a glass of milk for a definitive solace treat.

Cheesecake:

Cheesecake is a rich and smooth sweet that comes in different flavors and styles. From New York-style cheesecake to fruity varieties like strawberry or lemon, there's a cheesecake for everybody. Top it with a natural product compote or chocolate ganache for added guilty pleasure.

Banana Split:

A tomfoolery and nostalgic sweet, the banana split is a genuine group pleaser. It includes a split banana finished off with scoops of frozen yogurt (frequently vanilla, chocolate, and strawberry), hot fudge or chocolate sauce, whipped cream, nuts, and a clincher. A great treat's ideally suited for sharing.

These are only a couple of instances of the innumerable sweet recipes out there. Whether you favor something rich and chocolatey or light and fruity, there's a treat recipe to fulfill your sweet tooth. Analyze in the kitchen, attempt new flavors, and feel free to get imaginative with your pastries. All things considered, treat is the ideal chance to enjoy and partake in the better things throughout everyday life.

Quick Berry Parfait

Speedy Berry Parfait: A Superb and Sound Treat

Assuming that you're looking for a reviving and nutritious treat that can be prepared in no time, look no farther than the Speedy Berry Parfait. Overflowing with the dynamic kinds of new berries and layered with smooth yogurt, this brilliant treat is ideal for any event, whether it's a relaxed evening nibble or a rich finale to an evening gathering.

To simplify this yet impeccable pastry, you'll require only a small bunch of fixings:

New Berries: Pick your number one variety of berries, like strawberries, blueberries, raspberries, or blackberries. Choose occasional assortments to partake in the pinnacle of their normal pleasantness and deliciousness.

Greek Yogurt: The rich and tart nature of Greek yogurt gives the ideal equilibrium to the pleasantness of the berries. It's likewise loaded with protein and probiotics, making it a better option in contrast to customary cream-based treats.

Honey or Maple Syrup: A sprinkle of regular sugar like honey or maple syrup improves the general flavor profile of the parfait. Change the sum as indicated by your inclination for pleasantness.

Granola or Nuts (discretionary): For an additional crunch and surface, consider integrating some granola or squashed nuts of your decision. This step is discretionary however enthusiastically prescribed for those hoping to raise their parfait experience.

Presently, we should jump into the straightforward arrangement steps:

Wash the berries: Flush the new berries under chilly water and tenderly wipe them off with a paper towel. Eliminate any stems or leaves as needs be.

Set up the yogurt: In a bowl, join the Greek yogurt with a limited quantity of honey or maple syrup. Mix well to guarantee the sugar is equitably circulated all through the yogurt. Taste and change the pleasantness if necessary.

Layer the parfait: In a glass or pastry dish, begin by spooning a layer of the improved yogurt at the base. Then, add a layer of berries on top of the yogurt. Rehash this interaction, shifting back and forth among yogurt and berries, until the glass or dish is filled.

Embellish with garnishes (discretionary): Whenever wanted, sprinkle some granola or squashed nuts on the highest layer of the parfait. This adds a magnificent crunch and an additional bit of flavor.

Furthermore, presto! Your Fast Berry Parfait is fit to be delighted in. The mix of succulent berries, rich yogurt, and discretionary crunchy garnishes makes a tasty ensemble of surfaces and tastes. It's a righteous extravagance that fulfills your sweet tooth while sustaining your body with fundamental supplements.

Go ahead and try different things with various varieties of this parfait by consolidating different natural products, like cut bananas or diced mangoes, or by adding a sprinkle of citrus zing for a zingy curve. The conceivable outcomes are unfathomable, permitting you to fit the sweet to your own inclinations and occasional accessibility.

Serve the Fast Berry Parfait chilled and relish each spoonful, appreciating the explosion of flavors and the difference of surfaces. Whether delighted in alone or imparted to friends and family, this straightforward and sound treat makes certain to turn into a most loved go-to dessert in your culinary collection.

Chocolate Mug Cake

A chocolate mug cake is a wonderful and simple to-make treat that fulfills your desires for a warm and gooey pastry. A solitary serving pastry can be ready in only a couple of moments utilizing straightforward fixings and a microwave. The magnificence of a chocolate mug cake lies in its effortlessness and the way that you can partake in a newly heated cake without the requirement for a broiler or broad planning.

To make a chocolate mug cake, you will require a couple of essential fixings that are generally tracked down in many kitchens. These incorporate regular flour, sugar, unsweetened cocoa powder, baking powder, milk, vegetable oil, and a spot of salt. You can likewise add additional items like chocolate chips, vanilla concentrate, or a bit of Nutella for added character.

The method involved with making a chocolate mug cake is unquestionably clear. Begin by whisking together the dry fixings in a microwave-safe mug or a little bowl. This guarantees that the fixings are uniformly appropriated. Then, add the wet fixings like milk, vegetable oil, and vanilla concentrate to the dry blend, and mix until you have a smooth player. Assuming you decide to add chocolate chips or some other additional items, crease them into the hitter at this stage.

When your hitter is prepared, pop the mug into the microwave and cook on high for around one to two minutes. The cooking time might fluctuate relying upon the wattage of your microwave, so it's smart to watch out for it. The cake will rise and become cushy as it cooks. Be careful not to overcook it, as it might become dry.

While the concocting time is, cautiously eliminate the mug from the microwave (it will be hot!) and let it cool briefly. You can partake in the cake straightforwardly from the mug or delicately slide it onto a plate for a more stylish show. You can likewise add a sprinkle of powdered sugar, a bit of whipped cream, or a scoop of frozen yogurt on top to take your chocolate mug cake to a higher degree of flavor.

The outcome is a warm, damp, and debauched chocolate cake with a fudgy surface. The smell of chocolate swirls all around as you take your most memorable nibble, and the rich, extreme flavor will leave you hankering for more. Best of all, you can enjoy this awesome treat at whatever point the mind-set strikes you, as it requires negligible exertion and investment to prepare.

Chocolate mug cakes are ideally suited for fulfilling unexpected pastry desires, yet they can likewise be a tomfoolery and simple action to do with kids. You can include them during the time spent estimating and blending the fixings, permitting them to encounter the delight of making their own heavenly pastry.

Whether you are a chocolate sweetheart searching for a convenient solution or somebody who needs to take a shot at a straightforward baking recipe, a chocolate mug cake is a phenomenal decision. A wonderful treat brings moment satisfaction and permits you to partake in the consoling decency of a custom made cake in simply an issue of minutes.

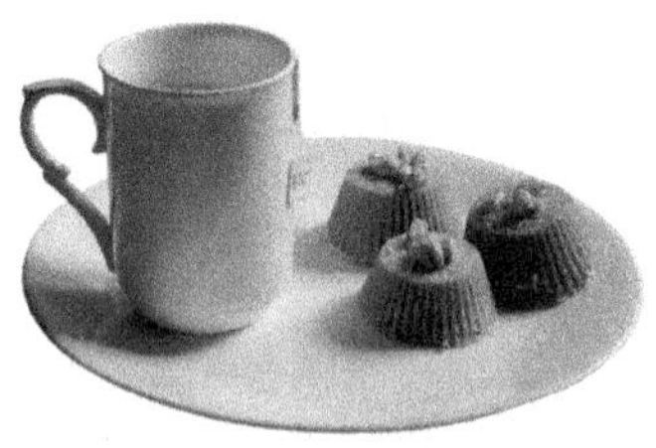

Frozen Banana Bites

Frozen banana nibbles are a superb and solid treat that joins the normal pleasantness of bananas with the smoothness of chocolate and the smash of different garnishes. They are not difficult to endlessly make for an ideal tidbit or sweet choice, particularly during warm climate.

To plan frozen banana chomps, you will require ready bananas, chocolate, and various garnishes. Here is a straightforward recipe to kick you off:

Fixings:

Ready bananas

Dim or drain chocolate (or your favored chocolate sort)

Fixings of your decision (e.g., slashed nuts, destroyed coconut, sprinkles, squashed treats, and so on.)

Popsicle sticks or toothpicks

Directions:

Strip the bananas and cut them into reduced down pieces, around 1-2 inches long.

Embed a popsicle stick or toothpick into every banana piece. This will make it simpler to deal with and plunge them later.

Line a baking sheet or plate with material paper.

Soften the chocolate in a microwave-safe bowl or utilizing a twofold heater on the burner. Mix infrequently until smooth and totally liquefied.

Plunge every banana piece into the dissolved chocolate, ensuring it's completely covered. You can utilize a spoon or fork to assist with the plunging system, guaranteeing the chocolate covers the banana equally.

When you've plunged a banana piece, roll it in your picked garnishes while the chocolate is as yet wet. This will assist the garnishes with sticking to the banana.

Put the covered banana nibbles on the lined baking sheet or plate and rehash the interaction until all the banana pieces are covered and beaten.

Whenever you've wrapped up covering all the banana chomps, place the baking sheet or plate in the cooler.

Permit the banana chomps to freeze for somewhere around 2-3 hours, or until totally strong.

Once frozen, move the banana nibbles to an impenetrable compartment or ziplock pack for capacity in the cooler. They can be saved for a considerable length of time.

Frozen banana chomps offer a huge number of flavor blends. You can try different things with various garnishes to suit your taste inclinations. For an exemplary mix, have a go at garnish them with slashed nuts like peanuts, almonds, or pecans. In the event that you partake in the tropical flavors, destroyed coconut or dried pineapple could be an extraordinary decision.

Sprinkles or squashed treats can add a tomfoolery and vivid touch.

These frozen treats are flavorful as well as give a few medical advantages. Bananas are a rich wellspring of potassium, L-ascorbic acid, and dietary fiber. Dull chocolate, with some restraint, offers cell reinforcements and may advance heart wellbeing. By picking better garnishes like nuts or dried natural products, you can additionally improve their healthy benefit.

Frozen banana nibbles are a flexible and invigorating pastry or bite that can be delighted in by individuals, all things considered. Whether you're searching for a virtuous treat or an innovative method for integrating more natural product into your eating regimen, these wonderful frozen treats make certain to fulfill your sweet tooth.

Conclusion

All in all, six-minute feasts offer a helpful and productive answer for people with occupied timetables or restricted opportunity to get ready food. These dinners are intended to be speedy and simple to make, permitting individuals to partake in a fantastic feast without going through hours in the kitchen.

One of the vital advantages of six-minute dinners is their effortlessness. With only a couple of essential fixings and insignificant cooking time, anybody can make a nutritious and tasty dish. These dinners frequently center around utilizing new and healthy fixings, making them a better option in contrast to handled and pre-bundled feasts.

Moreover, six-minute feasts can be modified to fit individual inclinations and dietary limitations. Whether you're a veggie lover, vegetarian, or have explicit sensitivities, there are various recipes accessible that take special care of different dietary necessities. This flexibility considers a different scope of feasts that can be delighted in by individuals with various preferences and necessities.

The efficient part of six-minute feasts couldn't possibly be more significant. In the present high speed world, carving out opportunity to cook can be a test. In any case, with these speedy and simple recipes, people can in any case partake in a home-prepared feast without forfeiting important time. This is especially useful for the people who need to focus on their wellbeing and prosperity yet have restricted chance to devote to cooking.

Besides, the comfort of six-minute dinners reaches out past cooking time. These feasts frequently require negligible cleanup, with less pots, dish, and utensils to wash. This can be a critical benefit for the people who need to smooth out their cooking cycle and lessen the time spent on kitchen-related errands.

While six-minute feasts offer many benefits, it's essential to take note of that they may not necessarily in all cases give the very profundity of flavor and intricacy as dishes that call for greater investment and work to plan. Notwithstanding, they act as a commonsense answer for people looking for speedy, scrumptious, and nutritious dinners.

All in all, six-minute feasts are an important asset for occupied people searching for a period effective method for planning dinners without settling on taste and nourishment. They offer effortlessness, customization, and comfort, making them an extraordinary choice for the people who need to eat well without going through hours in the kitchen. Integrating six-minute dinners into your cooking routine can assist you with keeping a solid way of life and give you additional opportunity to zero in on different parts of your life.

Enjoying Quick and Delicious Meals

In the present speedy world, carving out opportunity to get ready and partake in a delightful feast can frequently be a test. Notwithstanding, it doesn't mean you need to forfeit flavor or settle for undesirable choices. With a touch of arranging and innovativeness, you can in any case appreciate fast and delightful feasts that fulfill your taste buds and sustain your body.

Here are a few hints to assist you with getting a charge out of speedy and heavenly dinners:

Feast arranging: Invest an energy every week to design your dinners ahead of time. This permits you to make a shopping list and guarantees you have every one of the important fixings close by. Search for recipes that are speedy and simple to plan, or consider cluster preparing and feast preparing to save time during the week.

One-pot ponders: Embrace the straightforwardness of one-pot dinners. These dishes frequently require insignificant arrangement and cleanup while as yet conveying awesome flavors. Whether it's a good soup, a tasty sautéed food, or an encouraging pasta dish, one-pot feasts can be an efficient arrangement without compromising taste.

Keep a very much supplied storeroom: Having an all around loaded storage room is fundamental for fast and scrumptious feasts. Try to have staple fixings like grains (rice, quinoa), canned beans, pasta, canned tomatoes, flavors, and sauces. These things can act as the establishment for some speedy and delicious dishes.

Use alternate routes: Exploit efficient easy routes like pre-cut vegetables, pre-cooked proteins (like rotisserie chicken or canned fish), or frozen leafy foods. These accommodation things can essentially decrease planning time while as yet giving phenomenal flavor and sustenance.

Explore different avenues regarding flavors: Feel free to attempt new flavor blends and examination with flavors and spices. They can change even the least difficult dish into a culinary joy. Investigate various foods and cooking methods to keep your dinners intriguing and invigorating.

Speedy and solid bites: When you're in a rush, it's enticing to go after unfortunate tidbits. All things considered, stock your kitchen with fast and solid choices like new natural products, pre-cut vegetables with hummus or Greek yogurt plunge, nuts, or hand crafted energy balls. These tidbits will keep you fulfilled and empowered until your next dinner.

Utilize kitchen devices: Put resources into kitchen contraptions that can make your cooking cycle more productive. Apparatuses like tension cookers, slow cookers, air fryers, or food processors can assist you with getting ready feasts rapidly and without any problem. They can save you time and exertion while as yet delivering tasty outcomes.

Get inventive with extras: Don't allow extras to go to squander. All things considered, reuse them into new feasts or use them as parts for speedy and simple dishes. For instance, extra broiled chicken can be transformed into a delightful chicken plate of mixed greens, or cooked grains can be changed into a scrumptious grain bowl with new vegetables and a delectable dressing.

Keep in mind, getting a charge out of speedy and heavenly dinners doesn't need to be a test. With a touch of arranging, imagination, and some efficient procedures, you can relish tasty dishes that sustain your body and give pleasure as you would prefer buds. So feel free to investigate the universe of speedy and tasty cooking!

Importance of Balancing Convenience and Nutrition

Adjusting comfort and nourishment is essential for keeping a solid way of life in the present speedy world. In our cutting edge society, we frequently end up shuffling different obligations, which can prompt time requirements and a dependence on speedy and helpful food choices. Be that as it may, it is vital to perceive the meaning of focusing on sustenance close by comfort to guarantee our general prosperity. Comfort assumes a huge part in our food decisions. Drive-through joints, prepared to-eat dinners, and handled snacks have become progressively predominant because of their simplicity of availability and efficient nature. While these choices might offer comfort, they frequently miss the mark on supplements and are high in unfortunate fixings like added sugars, undesirable fats, and unnecessary sodium. Depending too vigorously on these accommodation food sources can prompt different medical problems like weight, coronary illness, and supplement lacks.

Then again, nourishment is essential for keeping up with ideal wellbeing and prosperity. An even eating routine that incorporates different entire food sources gives the essential supplements, nutrients, and minerals our bodies need to appropriately work. Legitimate nourishment upholds resistant capability, helps with weight the executives, further develops energy levels, and lessens the gamble of ongoing sicknesses. By focusing on sustenance, we can upgrade our general personal satisfaction and further develop our drawn out wellbeing results.

Finding the harmony among comfort and nourishment is the way to embracing a reasonable and sound way of life. Here are a few methodologies to accomplish this equilibrium:

Dinner arranging: Distributing time to design and plan feasts ahead of time can assist with finding some kind of harmony among accommodation and sustenance. This permits you to pick better fixings and control segment sizes, while as yet saving time during occupied periods.

Solid in a hurry choices: Search out better comfort food sources, for example, pre-cut products of the soil, yogurt cups, or entire grain tidbits, that give fundamental supplements without compromising comfort. These choices are promptly accessible in numerous stores and can be extraordinary options in contrast to unfortunate cheap food or handled snacks.

Cooking in bunches: Planning bigger amounts of feasts and freezing them in individual bits can be a period effective method for having nutritious dinners promptly accessible when time is restricted. This approach guarantees you have solid choices close by, decreasing the compulsion to decide on less nutritious decisions.

Careful eating: It is fundamental to be aware of what and how we eat, in any event, when comfort takes need. Dial back, relish your food, and focus on segment sizes. By rehearsing careful eating, you can pursue better decisions and try not to revel in advantageous yet less nutritious choices.

Instruction and mindfulness: Remain educated about nourishment and the effect regarding your food decisions on your wellbeing. Foster a comprehension of essential nourishing standards, read food marks, and know about the fixings in the food sources you devour. This information enables you to go with informed choices that focus on sustenance, even notwithstanding comfort.

Accomplishing a harmony among comfort and sustenance is generally difficult, yet it is an interest in your drawn out wellbeing and prosperity. By settling on cognizant decisions and tracking down inventive ways of integrating nutritious food sources into your bustling way of life, you can figure out some kind of harmony that upholds your general wellbeing objectives. Keep in mind, little changes and careful decisions can have a massive effect in the manner you support your body and lead a sound, satisfying life.